# 31 Days of Encouragement

By Karen V. Martin

This book is dedicated to my husband, Lawrence.
Thank you for being my earthly rock and inspiration.

# Table of Contents

# The Cost of Disobedience

In the beginning, God created man to have verbal communion with him. Everything God created He gave to man the freedom to enjoy; except for one. Of that one, God gave a command: "you shall not...." However, staying true to our sinful nature, man disobeyed God's command, and communion with God was broken, creating a separation between God and man.

That one act of disobedience by one man was inherited by all mankind. But, God in His infinite wisdom, in advance, prepared a plan of redemption for us, beginning with Abraham.

Jesus Christ, being obedient unto death, rescued us from eternal death, and restored us to a right relationship with Almighty God. The disobedience of one man brought death, but the obedience of one Man brought life eternal.


## Today's Readings

**Genesis 2:16-17**

*And the Lord God commanded the man, "You are free to eat from any tree in the garden; but you must not eat from the tree of the knowledge of good and evil, for when you eat from it you will certainly die."*

**Genesis 17:4-5**

*"As for me, this is my covenant with you: You will be the father of many nations. No longer will you be called Abram; your name will be Abraham, for I have made you a father of many nations.*

**1 Corinthians 15:22**

*For as in Adam all die, so also in Christ shall all be made alive.*

**John 3:15-16**

*...that everyone who believes may have eternal life in him." For God so loved the world that he gave his one and only Son, that whoever believes in him shall not perish but have eternal life.*

# Children of Abraham

Abraham made mistakes, and failed several times.....however, he never stopped trusting, and believing in God. Abraham continually looked to God, obeyed, and waited on Him to bring to fruition that which He had promised - no matter how long it took. Because of that, God credited Abraham's faith as righteousness.

The moment we accepted Jesus Christ by faith; believing in our hearts, and confessing Him to be the Son of God, we became children of Abraham. Therefore, as children of Abraham, we are also heirs to the promise made to Abraham. What a blessing.

### Today's Readings

**Genesis 17:5-7**

*No longer will you be called Abram; your name will be Abraham, for I have made you a father of many nations. I will make you very fruitful; I will make nations of you, and kings will come from you. I will establish my covenant as an everlasting covenant between me and you and your descendants after you for the generations to come, to be your God and the God of your descendants after you.*

**Galatians 3:7-9; 16; 26-29**

*Understand, then, that those who have faith are children of Abraham. Scripture foresaw that God would justify the Gentiles by faith, and announced the gospel in advance to Abraham: "All nations will be blessed through you." So those who rely on faith are blessed along with Abraham, the man of faith.*

*The promises were spoken to Abraham and to his seed. Scripture does not say "and to seeds," meaning many people, but "and to your seed," meaning one person, who is Christ.*

*So in Christ Jesus you are all children of God through faith, for all of you who were baptized into Christ have clothed yourselves with Christ. There is neither Jew nor Gentile, neither slave nor free, nor is there male and female, for you are all one in Christ Jesus. If you belong to Christ, then you are Abraham's seed, and heirs according to the promise.*

# When We Believe

When we believe in Jesus Christ, two wonderful things happen:

First, every sin we have committed are given to Jesus Christ; and second, we receive forgiveness, and is made right with Almighty God once and for all time – nothing can change that.

This exchange is a free gift from God, it cannot be earned; we cannot work for it. We just have to believe and accept the gift, which is attainable only through Christ Jesus.

## Today's Readings

**Romans 6:23**
> *For the wages of sin is death, but the gift of God is eternal life in Christ Jesus our Lord.*

**Ephesians 2: 8-9**
> *For by grace you have been saved through faith, and that not of yourselves; it is the gift of God, not of works, lest anyone should boast.*

# The Question Is

Accepting God's free gift of eternal life through Jesus Christ makes us eternally secure in Him. And while we may be secure in Him, we are still humans living in a sinful world; as such, we will also feel the pressures, and temptations, of sin. However, because we have God's Holy Spirit living within us, we have the power we need to walk away from sin by the grace of God.

The question is: when faced with the temptation to sin, will you choose to walk away, or will you choose to ignore God's Holy Spirit, and give in to temptation?

## Today's Readings

**2 Corinthians 12:9**

> *But he said to me, "My grace is sufficient for you, for my power is made perfect in weakness." Therefore I will boast all the more gladly about my weaknesses, so that Christ's power may rest on me.*

**Philippians 4:13**

> *I can do all this through him who gives me strength.*

**Ephesians 6:10**

> *Finally, be strong in the Lord and in the strength of his might.*

**Colossians 1:11**

> *May you be strengthened with all power, according to his glorious might, for all endurance and patience with joy,*

**Ephesians 3:16**

> *that according to the riches of his glory he may grant you to be strengthened with power through his Spirit in your inner being*

# Newness of Life

Jesus Christ was beaten, insulted, spat on, and nailed to a cross in our place – yours and mine. Everything we (you and I) have done, or will ever do, was nailed to that cross with Him. When He was buried, He took all our sins and transgressions down to the grave with Him, leaving us free, forgiven, and pardoned. On the day Christ rose from the dead, we (you and I) by the glory of God, rose with Him to walk in newness of life; eternal life.

Therefore, the person we used to be no longer exists. We became new creations in Christ the day we believed, and accepted Him as our Savior. It was by God's grace, mercy and love that He granted us this free gift. We did not work for it; we've done nothing to earn it (Titus 3:5-7).

So, we should choose daily to walk in obedience to our Heavenly Father without murmuring, or complaining, regardless of our circumstances. Remember, He who called us is faithful.

## Today's Readings

### Romans 6:3-4

*Or don't you know that all of us who were baptized into Christ Jesus were baptized into his death? We were therefore buried with him through baptism into death in order that, just as Christ was raised from the dead through the glory of the Father, we too may live a new life.*

### Colossians 2:12-14

*having been buried with him in baptism, in which you were also raised with him through your faith in the working of God, who raised him from the dead. When you were dead in your sins and in the uncircumcision of your flesh, God made you alive with Christ. He forgave us all our sins, having canceled the charge of our legal indebtedness, which stood against us and condemned us; he has taken it away, nailing it to the cross.*

# Under Grace

The truth is, because of what Jesus Christ did at Calvary, we have been given the glorious opportunity to become different people from what we use to be – spiritually, emotionally, mentally, and psychologically. Jesus gave it all up so we would no longer be slaves to sin, walking in darkness; but instead be slaves to righteousness, walking in His marvelous Light.

That being said, there are two undeniable truths we must always remember:  death is the payment, the penalty, for everyone who continues to deny Christ, and walk in sin; but eternal life is the free gift for everyone who believes in Jesus Christ, and accepts Him as their Lord and Savior.

### Today's Readings

**Romans 6:14**
> *For sin shall no longer be your master, because you are not under the law, but under grace.*

**Romans 6:23**
> *For the wages of sin is death, but the gift of God is eternal life in Christ Jesus our Lord.*

**Ephesians 2:8**
> *For it is by grace you have been saved, through faith—and this is not from yourselves, it is the gift of God*

**Colossians 1:13-14**
> *For he has rescued us from the dominion of darkness and brought us into the kingdom of the Son he loves, in whom we have redemption, the forgiveness of sins.*

# Our All In All

For in Him (Jesus Christ) we live, and move, and have our being (Acts 17:28).

In Him we have life. Everything that we are, and can be, is wrapped up in Jesus Christ. He is our strength in the storm; our courage when we face our foe; our peace and defense in the valley; our comfort when we are broken. He gives us boldness and strength to stand; He sustains us to persevere. When we cannot take another step, He moves for us; when we have lost the will to go on, He revives us; and when we get to the brink, He pulls us back. He is our everything, and apartment from Him we are nothing, can do nothing.

Matthew Henry puts it this way:

> *"We are his offspring, He is our Father, and since we live in Him, we should live for Him; since we move in Him, we should move toward Him; since we have our being in Him, we should consecrate our lives to Him."*

And all of God's children say, Amen!!

## Today's Readings

**Genesis 2:7**
> *Then the Lord God formed a man from the dust of the ground and breathed into his nostrils the breath of life, and the man became a living being.*

**Job 12:10**
> *In his hand is the life of every creature and the breath of all mankind.*

**John 15:5**

*"I am the vine; you are the branches. If you remain in me and I in you, you will bear much fruit; apart from me you can do nothing.*

**Romans 8:11**

*And if the Spirit of him who raised Jesus from the dead is living in you, he who raised Christ from the dead will also give life to your mortal bodies because of his Spirit who lives in you.*

# Final and Complete

We are God's children; His creations. He is undoubtedly the Creator. He created the world and everything in it, which means everything belongs to Him. God gave life to each of us, He gave us thought. We move and have our being because of Him; therefore, the created cannot exist without the Creator.

We have absolutely nothing that God wants. He is not something we (the created) made ourselves to worship. No, He was not designed, crafted, or molded by man, so that He can be kept in a box, in a temple, or in a particular place to be manipulated, and shaped to our every will and desires.

He is the Lord God Almighty, the Creator of this universe. When we believe in Jesus Christ, His Holy Spirit comes and lives within our hearts, so that wherever we are, whatever we're doing, He is right there with us. He promised to never leave us, nor forsake us, and God can do everything and anything, except this……..He cannot lie. So, if He said he will never leave us, it is so; and that makes it final and complete for me.

## Today's Readings

**Genesis 1:27**

> *So God created mankind in his own image, in the image of God he created them; male and female he created them.*

**Acts 17:29**

> *"Therefore since we are God's offspring, we should not think that the divine being is like gold or silver or stone— an image made by human design and skill.*

**Hebrews 13:5**

*Keep your lives free from the love of money and be content with what you have, because God has said, "Never will I leave you; never will I forsake you."*

# You Are Not Alone

As children of God, His Holy Spirit sustains, and carries us through whatever trials and tribulations we may go through. As such, because the Holy Spirit lives within us, when we are wronged, persecuted, and/or face tribulations, it is not just to us (the individual) that the wrong is being done; it is also being done to God's Holy Spirit.

Consequently, we must be very careful how we treat each other, because it is not just the individual we are interacting with, but also Jesus Christ, through His Holy Spirit who dwells in each child of God. When we treat each other with disrespect, abuse, slander, etc., it is also Christ we are treating in that manner.

Incidentally, this principle applies even more so in the relationship between husbands and wives. We are first and foremost children of God, and therefore brothers and sisters in faith; thus, it holds true that we treat each other accordingly.

### Today's Readings

**Acts 9:3-6**

*As he neared Damascus on his journey, suddenly a light from heaven flashed around him. He fell to the ground and heard a voice say to him, "Saul, Saul, why do you persecute me?" "Who are you, Lord?" Saul asked. "I am Jesus, whom you are persecuting," he replied.*

**Ephesians 5:29-30**

*In this same way, husbands ought to love their wives as their own bodies. He who loves his wife loves himself. After all, no one ever hated their own body, but they feed*

*and care for their body, just as Christ does the church—*
*for we are members of his body.*

**Matthew 25:40**
  *"The King will reply, 'Truly I tell you, whatever you did*
*for one of the least of these brothers and sisters of mine,*
*you did for me.'*

# You Are Not Your Own

Sometimes we go through difficult situations in life that threaten to take us out, but by the grace of God. Those difficulties may be because of no fault of our own, bad decisions, consequences of choices we've made, or just simply because of our disobedience to God. Regardless of the reason for the difficulties, as children of God, He can use those said difficulties for His purpose, and for our good.

God has called each of His children for a purpose, and sometimes we may have to go through "the fire" in order for us to be prepared for that purpose. Just as gold must go through the fire to be refined, so must the child of God in order for us to be a vessel ready for His use. We are not our own; we belong to God, and therefore His to do with as He so chooses.

### Today's Readings

**Romans 8:28**

> *And we know that for those who love God all things work together for good, for those who are called according to his purpose.*

**James 1:12**

> *Blessed is the man who remains steadfast under trial, for when he has stood the test he will receive the crown of life, which God has promised to those who love him.*

**1 Peter 5:10**

> *And after you have suffered a little while, the God of all grace, who has called you to his eternal glory in Christ, will himself restore, confirm, strengthen, and establish you.*

**Acts 9:15-16**

> *But the Lord said to Ananias, "Go! This man is my chosen instrument to proclaim my name to the Gentiles and their kings and to the people of Israel. 16 I will show him how much he must suffer for my name."*

# Nothing Means Nothing

When we accepted Jesus Christ as our personal Lord and Savior, we were pardoned of all of our sins. We are no longer considered enemies of God, but are now His forgiven children. Jesus' sacrifice paid the penalty for us to be reconciled to God for all eternity.

Consequently, once we believed, nothing in all of creation, and beyond, can ever separate us from the love of God: "neither death nor life, neither angels nor demons, neither the present nor the future, nor any powers, neither height nor depth, nor anything else in all creation, will be able to separate us from the love of God….," Romans 8:38-39.

Did you get that? Nothing means just that, nothing. The day you believed, you became His child, and *nothing* can ever change that. Get it, receive it, believe it.

### Today's Readings

**Romans 5:6-11**

*You see, at just the right time, when we were still powerless, Christ died for the ungodly. Very rarely will anyone die for a righteous person, though for a good person someone might possibly dare to die. But God demonstrates his own love for us in this: While we were still sinners, Christ died for us.*

*Since we have now been justified by his blood, how much more shall we be saved from God's wrath through him! For if, while we were God's enemies, we were reconciled to him through the death of his Son, how much more, having been reconciled, shall we be saved through his life!*

*Not only is this so, but we also boast in God through our Lord Jesus Christ, through whom we have now received reconciliation.*

### Romans 8:37-39

*No, in all these things we are more than conquerors through him who loved us. For I am convinced that neither death nor life, neither angels nor demons, neither the present nor the future, nor any powers, neither height nor depth, nor anything else in all creation, will be able to separate us from the love of God that is in Christ Jesus our Lord.*

# The Importance of Quiet Times

One of the most beautiful things about having a relationship with Jesus Christ, is the peace and sustaining you feel regardless of the trials, or tribulations, you may be experiencing. No one can live an obedient/devotional life 24/7; however, it is the sincere daily pursuit of it that makes a difference. God knows our hearts, so there is no faking it.

Daily conversation with Jesus Christ is a vital part of being a Christian. It is a two-way thing: first, it brings us closer to God; and second, it opens our hearts to hear, and understand, what He has to impart to us. It is in those quiet times of conversations with God that He strengthens, and guides us through our life's journey – stormy or calm.

## Today's Readings

**Acts 15:8**

*God, who knows the heart, showed that he accepted them by giving the Holy Spirit to them, just as he did to us.*

**Hebrews 4:13**

*Nothing in all creation is hidden from God's sight. Everything is uncovered and laid bare before the eyes of him to whom we must give account.*

# More Than

It is not a person's station in life (rich or poor), nor their birth position, nor their nationality, nor the color of their skin that matters to God. It is the fear of God, and the content and desires of the heart that matters to Him.

It is how they live their lives for God: righteously, prayerfully, charitably to the best of their ability through God's Holy Spirit. Being a "good person," or doing "good deeds" amounts to nothing without faith in Jesus Christ, our Lord.

## Today's Readings

**Deuteronomy 10:17**

*For the Lord your God is God of gods and Lord of lords, the great God, mighty and awesome, who shows no partiality and accepts no bribes.*

**Acts 10:34-35**

*Then Peter began to speak: "I now realize how true it is that God does not show favoritism but accepts from every nation the one who fears him and does what is right.*

**Galatians 2:6**

*As for those who were held in high esteem—whatever they were makes no difference to me; God does not show favoritism—they added nothing to my message.*

**Colossians 3:11**

*Here there is no Gentile or Jew, circumcised or uncircumcised, barbarian, Scythian, slave or free, but Christ is all, and is in all.*

# The Chains That Bind

Unfortunately, in this life some of us are bound by chains. No, not physical chains; emotional, mental and spiritual chains caused by decisions or choices we have made, or of no fault of our own making. In some instances, it may seem like those chains are impossible to break; however, by submitting our hearts and will to God, He can break those chains and set us free.

As we immerse ourselves in His Word, He will revive us to a new revelation, and instructs us how to get up, gird ourselves with the belt of truth, and walk in the sandals of peace. As we put on the cloak of His Holy Spirit and follow Him, He will take us *through*, and deliver us out of our troubles, even those that seemed impossible.

His power is certainly not limited, so nothing is impossible for our God.

### Today's Readings

**Numbers 11:23**
> *And the Lord said to Moses, "Is the Lord's hand shortened? Now you shall see whether my word will come true for you or not."*

**Jeremiah 32:27**
> *"Behold, I am the Lord, the God of all flesh. Is anything too hard for me?*

**Job 42:2**
> *"I know that you can do all things, and that no purpose of yours can be thwarted.*

**Matthew 19:26**

*But Jesus looked at them and said, "With man this is impossible, but with God all things are possible."*

**Ephesians 3:20**

*Now to him who is able to do far more abundantly than all that we ask or think, according to the power at work within us,*

## Prayer

To You, Heavenly Father, we release our will, asking for your forgiven, your deliverance, and your blessing, in Jesus' name. Amen.

# Afterwards

For some of us, when we have been delivered from our "chains," the tendency is to fall away from following God with that fervency and determination we did when we needed His deliverance; but, the opposite should be true. It is after our deliverance that we should follow Him in earnest, and faithfulness.

His deliverance is sure, and what He has put in place for us, no one can displace. Doors that He has opened no one can close. So, when we come to the realization of what God has done for us, our commitment, our allegiance, our reverence, our determination should be to Him, and to serve Him with our lives until He returns for us.

## Today's Readings

**Acts 12:9-11**

> *Peter followed him out of the prison, but he had no idea that what the angel was doing was really happening; he thought he was seeing a vision. They passed the first and second guards and came to the iron gate leading to the city. It opened for them by itself, and they went through it. When they had walked the length of one street, suddenly the angel left him. Then Peter came to himself and said, "Now I know without a doubt that the Lord has sent his angel and rescued me from Herod's clutches and from everything the Jewish people were hoping would happen."*

**Daniel 3:28**

> *Nebuchadnezzar answered and said, "Blessed be the God of Shadrach, Meshach, and Abednego, who has sent his angel and delivered his servants, who trusted in him, and*

*set aside the king's command, and yielded up their bodies rather than serve and worship any god except their own God.*

**Psalm 34:7**

*The angel of the Lord encamps around those who fear him, and delivers them.*

# It Really Wasn't Your Doing

When God uses us to accomplish something, we should be very careful that we do not take credit for that accomplishment. Likewise, when God uses someone to bless, or fulfill a need for us, we should be ever so careful how we show our appreciation to that someone whom GOD used to fulfill His purpose for us.

In everything, the glory and praise of God must never be given to man; and man must never claim the glory and praise of God for himself. It really wasn't your doing.


## Today's Readings

### Acts 14:13-14

*The priest of Zeus, whose temple was just outside the city, brought bulls and wreaths to the city gates because he and the crowd wanted to offer sacrifices to them. But when the apostles Barnabas and Paul heard of this, they tore their clothes and rushed out into the crowd, shouting: "Friends, why are you doing this? We too are only human, like you. We are bringing you good news, telling you to turn from these worthless things to the living God, who made the heavens and the earth and the sea and everything in them.*

### Acts 10:25-26

*When Peter entered, Cornelius met him and fell down at his feet and worshiped him. But Peter lifted him up, saying, "Stand up; I too am a man."*

### Acts 12:22-23

*They shouted, "This is the voice of a god, not of a man." Immediately, because Herod did not give praise to God, an*

32

*angel of the Lord struck him down, and he was eaten by worms and died.*

# By God's Grace Alone

No one can come to God unless He calls them. God is the One who opens our hearts to believe in His Son, Jesus Christ.

Because God is the One who calls us, and the One who opens our hearts to believe, no one can earn their salvation on their own accord; therefore, no one can brag, or boast, that it was their doing.

It is by God's grace, and God's grace alone that we are saved.

## Today's Readings

**Romans 8:28; 30**

> *And those he predestined, he also called; those he called, he also justified; those he justified, he also glorified.*

**1 Peter 2:9**

> *But you are a chosen people, a royal priesthood, a holy nation, God's special possession, that you may declare the praises of him who called you out of darkness into his wonderful light.*

**Acts 16:14**

> *One of those listening was a woman from the city of Thyatira named Lydia, a dealer in purple cloth. She was a worshiper of God. The Lord opened her heart to respond to Paul's message.*

**Luke 24:45**

> *Then he opened their minds so they could understand the Scriptures.*

**Ephesians 2:8-9**

*For it is by grace you have been saved, through faith—and this is not from yourselves, it is the gift of God; not by works, so that no one can boast.*

# Though He Slay Me

Job said, "Though He slays me, I will still praise Him," (Job 13:15).

Paul and Silas was humiliated, beaten, shackled, and thrown into prison for the truth. They had every reason to be angry, bitter, and resentful. Instead, they prayed and praised the Lord in spite of their circumstances. They even prayed for those who persecuted them. Because of their steadfast faith, God not only delivered them, He used their circumstances to accomplish His purposes for those around them.

Each of us will go through trials and tribulations at some point in our lives. When we do, as difficult as it may be, we should not murmur, complain or give up. Instead, we must remain steadfast, trusting, and believing in God. We should praise him *through* the circumstances; persevering and enduring in Him.

This same perseverance will build our character, which in turn will build our hope; hope in God. And that kind of hope will never disappoint us. Job, Paul, and Silas knew that. So should we.

### Today's Readings

**Acts 16:25-26**
> *About midnight Paul and Silas were praying and singing hymns to God, and the other prisoners were listening to them. Suddenly there was such a violent earthquake that the foundations of the prison were shaken. At once all the prison doors flew open, and everyone's chains came loose.*

**Romans 5:3-5**

*Not only so, but we also glory in our sufferings, because we know that suffering produces perseverance; perseverance, character; and character, hope. And hope does not put us to shame, because God's love has been poured out into our hearts through the Holy Spirit, who has been given to us.*

**James 1:2-3**

*Count it all joy, my brothers, when you meet trials of various kinds, for you know that the testing of your faith produces steadfastness.*

# Be Encouraged

When we go through difficult, or painful, situations we often asked, "why me?" or wonder if any good can come out of our difficulties. However, there are many instances in the word of God where He used difficult circumstances to accomplish His purpose for a particular individual, and for His people; such as Joseph, Daniel, Esther, Naomi, Job, Paul & Silas, to name a few.

If you are currently going through a difficult situation, be encouraged. Keep your eyes, heart, and mind on God. Though you may not see it, He can use your circumstances to achieve His purpose for you, your family, and for His people.

## Today's Readings

### Acts 16:22-34

*The crowd joined in the attack against Paul and Silas, and the magistrates ordered them to be stripped and beaten with rods. After they had been severely flogged, they were thrown into prison, and the jailer was commanded to guard them carefully. When he received these orders, he put them in the inner cell and fastened their feet in the stocks.*

*About midnight Paul and Silas were praying and singing hymns to God, and the other prisoners were listening to them. Suddenly there was such a violent earthquake that the foundations of the prison were shaken. At once all the prison doors flew open, and everyone's chains came loose. The jailer woke up, and when he saw the prison doors open, he drew his sword and was about to kill himself because he thought the prisoners had escaped. But Paul shouted, "Don't harm yourself! We are all here!"*

*The jailer called for lights, rushed in and fell trembling before Paul and Silas. He then brought them out and asked, "Sirs, what must I do to be saved?"*

*They replied, "Believe in the Lord Jesus, and you will be saved—you and your household." Then they spoke the word of the Lord to him and to all the others in his house. At that hour of the night the jailer took them and washed their wounds; then immediately he and all his household were baptized. The jailer brought them into his house and set a meal before them; he was filled with joy because he had come to believe in God—he and his whole household.*

# Know For Yourself

It is of utmost importance that we are vigilant in studying the word of God for ourselves, so we will be firm in what we know, and believe, about our faith, and most importantly, about Jesus Christ.

There are factions out there whose purpose it is to inject false teachings that sound so true that if we are not careful, we will believe them. Be extremely careful of people who claim that their interpretation of God's word is the correct interpretation, and that all other teachers' interpretation is incorrect. There is only one interpretation. Period.

Read for yourself, and ask the Holy Spirit to give you understanding. If what they tell you does not line up with the word of God, RUN in the opposite direction. Study for yourself, so you will know for yourself.

## Today's Readings

**2 Timothy 4:3**
> *For the time will come when people will not put up with sound doctrine. Instead, to suit their own desires, they will gather around them a great number of teachers to say what their itching ears want to hear.*

**Colossians 2:6-11**
> *Therefore, as you received Christ Jesus the Lord, so walk in him, rooted and built up in him and established in the faith, just as you were taught, abounding in thanksgiving. See to it that no one takes you captive by philosophy and empty deceit, according to human tradition, according to the elemental spirits of the world, and not according to*

*Christ. For in him the whole fullness of deity dwells bodily, and you have been filled in him, who is the head of all rule and authority.*

## 1 Timothy 6:3-5

*If anyone teaches otherwise and does not agree to the sound instruction of our Lord Jesus Christ and to godly teaching, they are conceited and understand nothing. They have an unhealthy interest in controversies and quarrels about words that result in envy, strife, malicious talk, evil suspicions and constant friction between people of corrupt mind, who have been robbed of the truth and who think that godliness is a means to financial gain.*

# Be Ever So Careful

As children of God, sometimes we say things without first stopping to think about what we're saying, or how it will affect those hearing it. Even worse, we behave as if what we say, or think for that matter, is concealed from Almighty God; but quite the contrary is true. God hears everything that proceeds out of our mouths, even that which is not spoken.

We must be careful that our response to trials and tribulations does not manifest itself in grumblings and complaints. Instead, we are to humbly trust God to see us through. Therefore, we ought to be ever so careful of what we speak about ourselves, about others, and especially what we say *to* others.

## Today's Readings

**Numbers 14:27-28**
> *"How long will this wicked community grumble against me? I have heard the complaints of these grumbling Israelites. So tell them, 'As surely as I live, declares the Lord, I will do to you the very thing I heard you say*

**James 3:5-6**
> *Likewise, the tongue is a small part of the body, but it makes great boasts. Consider what a great forest is set on fire by a small spark. The tongue also is a fire, a world of evil among the parts of the body. It corrupts the whole body, sets the whole course of one's life on fire, and is itself set on fire by hell.*

**James 3:8-12**
> *but no human being can tame the tongue. It is a restless evil, full of deadly poison. With the tongue we praise our*

42

*Lord and Father, and with it we curse human beings, who have been made in God's likeness. Out of the same mouth come praise and cursing. My brothers and sisters, this should not be. Can both fresh water and salt water flow from the same spring? My brothers and sisters, can a fig tree bear olives, or a grapevine bear figs? Neither can a salt spring produce fresh water.*

# Truth

Truth: what is it, and how do we attain it?

The dictionary renders the meaning of "truth" as, "the true or actual state of a matter;" "conformity with fact or reality;" and, "a verified or indisputable fact."

Truth is absolute; it is either black or white. There is one truth that all mankind needs to know: the truth about Jesus Christ.

The only way to know this truth for yourself is to spend time in the Word of God - the Bible. It is the verified, and indisputable truth about the birth, life, death, and bodily resurrection of our Lord and Savior, Jesus Christ.

Academic and intellectual knowledge is commendable, but, biblical knowledge is excellent. It is the one truth you will need for life's journey.

### Today's Readings

**John 8:31-32**
> ......*Jesus said, "If you hold to my teaching, you are really my disciples. Then you will know the truth, and the truth will set you free."*

**1 Corinthians 2:14**
> *The person without the Spirit does not accept the things that come from the Spirit of God but considers them foolishness, and cannot understand them because they are discerned only through the Spirit.*

**2 John 1:9**

> *Everyone who goes on ahead and does not abide in the teaching of Christ, does not have God. Whoever abides in the teaching has both the Father and the Son.*

**Hebrews 3:14**

> *For we have come to share in Christ, if indeed we hold our original confidence firm to the end.*

# Always There....Waiting

From one man God created the entire human race; all equal, none superior. He determined beforehand where each person would live, and the number of days set for each one of us to live. He is a God of purpose; a God of compassion; a God of grace and mercy; a God of great patience.

Though He has all power and might, and can make us do whatever He so chooses, He waits patiently for us to turn to Him of our own free will, out of our hunger for Him. He will never judge, never. He is always there....waiting.

## Today's Readings

**Acts 17:26-27**
> *From one man he made all the nations, that they should inhabit the whole earth; and he marked out their appointed times in history and the boundaries of their lands. God did this so that they would seek him and perhaps reach out for him and find him, though he is not far from any one of us.*

**Psalm 139:16**
> *Your eyes saw my unformed body; all the days ordained for me were written in your book before one of them came to be.*

**Isaiah 55:6**
> *Seek the Lord while he may be found; call on him while he is near.*

**Jeremiah 23:23-24**
> *"Am I only a God nearby," declares the Lord, "and not a God far away? Who can hide in secret places so that I*

*cannot see them?" declares the Lord. "Do not I fill heaven and earth?" declares the Lord.*

# Where Do You Stand?

There is coming a day when God will judge the world. He has set a day and time when all people will have to give an account for our actions, whether we believe in Him or not (Matthew 25:31-46). He created the world and everything in it; therefore, He has the right to judge it, the right to hold it accountable.

Knowing that day will come, God before hand, in His infinite wisdom, made provision for us. He made it possible for us to be forgiven, and freely gifted us with eternal life through His Son, Jesus Christ.

The shed blood of Christ made it possible for us to be pardoned of our sins, and be reconciled to God for all eternity. So....where do you stand?

### Today's Readings

**Acts 17: 30-31**

*In the past God overlooked such ignorance, but now he commands all people everywhere to repent. For he has set a day when he will judge the world with justice by the man he has appointed. He has given proof of this to everyone by raising him from the dead."*

**Roman 3:25**

*God presented Christ as a sacrifice of atonement, through the shedding of his blood—to be received by faith. He did this to demonstrate his righteousness, because in his forbearance he had left the sins committed beforehand unpunished—*

**Hebrews 9:28**

*so Christ was sacrificed once to take away the sins of many; and he will appear a second time, not to bear sin, but to bring salvation to those who are waiting for him.*

**1 John 4:10**

*This is love: not that we loved God, but that he loved us and sent his Son as an atoning sacrifice for our sins.*

# Unless He Wills It

God grants to each person "free will." We are free to do as we please...and, staying true to our nature, we do just that, forgetting that we are not our own. Forgetting that we belong to a mighty, sovereign God; forgetting that it is in Him we move, we breathe, and have our being.

Each day we make plans, doing all we know to do to see them succeed. There is nothing wrong with making plans; however, none of us is promised tomorrow. And unless it is God's will for us to see another day, those plans will not come to fruition.

Therefore, our thoughts at the beginning of each new day should be, "if God is willing, I will......."

## Today's Readings

**Acts 17:28**
> 'For in him we live and move and have our being.'[a] As some of your own poets have said, 'We are his offspring.'

**Acts 18:21**
> But as he left, he promised, "I will come back if it is God's will." Then he set sail from Ephesus.

**Romans 1:10**
> in my prayers at all times; and I pray that now at last by God's will the way may be opened for me to come to you.

**Hebrews 6:3**
> And God permitting, we will do so.

# In It But Not of It

Some of us who believe in Jesus Christ as Savior, and Lord, are still living in this world; but though we live in it, we are not of it. We belong to Almighty God. As such, how we live our lives as His children is a direct representation of Him.

For that reason, we must live our lives circumspectly for Him, as our lives are examples for others to follow, and we do not know who may be watching us; so, let's consecrate our lives for Him.

### Today's Readings

**Romans 2:21-24**
> *you, then, who teach others, do you not teach yourself? You who preach against stealing, do you steal? [22] You who say that people should not commit adultery, do you commit adultery? You who abhor idols, do you rob temples? [23] You who boast in the law, do you dishonor God by breaking the law?*

**Romans 12:2**
> *Do not conform to the pattern of this world, but be transformed by the renewing of your mind. Then you will be able to test and approve what God's will is—his good, pleasing and perfect will.*

**John 17:13-17**
> *"I am coming to you now, but I say these things while I am still in the world, so that they may have the full measure of my joy within them. 14 I have given them your word and the world has hated them, for they are not of the world any more than I am of the world. 15 My prayer is not that you take them out of the world but that you protect them from*

*the evil one. 16 They are not of the world, even as I am not of it. 17 Sanctify them by[d] the truth; your word is truth.*

# What Are You Looking For?

My encouragement for today is a very simple one. In John 1:38-39, two disciples heard Jesus spoke, and started following Him. Jesus turned to them and asked, "What do you seek?"

My questions for you today are: Who are you listening to? Who are you following? And, most importantly, "what are you looking for?"

Your answer can change the course of your life.

## Today's Readings

**John 1:38-39**

*Turning around, Jesus saw them following and asked, "What do you want?" They said, "Rabbi" (which means "Teacher"), "where are you staying?" "Come," he replied, "and you will see." So they went and saw where he was staying, and they spent that day with him. It was about four in the afternoon.*

**John 18:4**

*Then Jesus, knowing all that would happen to him, came forward and said to them, "Whom do you seek?"*

**John 18:7**

*So he asked them again, "Whom do you seek?" And they said, "Jesus of Nazareth."*

**Psalm 27:4**

*One thing have I asked of the Lord, that will I seek after: that I may dwell in the house of the Lord all the days of my life, to gaze upon the beauty of the Lord and to inquire in his temple.*

# Life Anew

Being born, physically, is the beginning of life. To be "born again" is to begin life anew spiritually. New nature; new beliefs; new principles; new affections; new aims; new desires; new understanding; new loyalties; and in some instances, new friends.

This new birth is life changing, life elevating, life sustaining, and is only attainable through belief in Jesus Christ, God's only Son.

Believing in Jesus Christ grants us access to the kingdom of our Sovereign God, and is available to anyone who calls on His name.

## Today's Readings

**John 3:3-5**

*Jesus replied, "Very truly I tell you, no one can see the kingdom of God unless they are born again." "How can someone be born when they are old?" Nicodemus asked. "Surely they cannot enter a second time into their mother's womb to be born!" Jesus answered, "Very truly I tell you, no one can enter the kingdom of God unless they are born of water and the Spirit.*

**Ezekiel 36:25-27**

*I will sprinkle clean water on you, and you will be clean; I will cleanse you from all your impurities and from all your idols. I will give you a new heart and put a new spirit in you; I will remove from you your heart of stone and give you a heart of flesh. And I will put my Spirit in you and*

*move you to follow my decrees and be careful to keep my
laws.*

## 2 Corinthians 5:17

*Therefore, if anyone is in Christ, he is a new creation. The
old has passed away; behold, the new has* come.

## 1 John 3:9

*No one born of God makes a practice of sinning, for God's
seed abides in him, and he cannot keep on sinning because
he has been born of God.*

# True Worship

True worship does not depend on a time or a place, or whether or not you are alone or in a group. True worship depends on the heart and mind, and the One they revere, and believe in. It is how we honor God in the way we live our lives, and how we treat each other.

Our Heavenly Father is to be worshipped anytime, and anywhere, with our total being (mind, body and soul) from a submissive and sincere heart.

## Today's Readings

**John 4:23-24**

*Yet a time is coming and has now come when the true worshipers will worship the Father in the Spirit and in truth, for they are the kind of worshipers the Father seeks. 24 God is spirit, and his worshipers must worship in the Spirit and in truth."*

**1 Samuel 12:24**

*Only fear the Lord and serve him faithfully with all your heart. For consider what great things he has done for you.*

**Romans 12:1**

*I appeal to you therefore, brothers, by the mercies of God, to present your bodies as a living sacrifice, holy and acceptable to God, which is your spiritual worship.*

**Hebrews 13:15-16**

*Through him then let us continually offer up a sacrifice of praise to God, that is, the fruit of lips that acknowledge his name.  Do not neglect to do good and to share what you have, for such sacrifices are pleasing to God.*

# Your Mess for His Best

Each of us has made decisions in our lives that may lead us to believe we can never be used by God to accomplish his purpose. Nonetheless, because He is from infinity to infinity; the beginning and the end; and everywhere in-between, He knew the entire story of our lives *before* He spoke this world into existence, still…..He loves us. He loves you.

Though you may have made a mess of things, your mess (and mine) does not surprise God. In fact, because He has called you for His purpose, He can use your mess to produce His best for you. His grace and His power know no limit.

## Today's Readings

**Psalm 139:16**

*Your eyes saw my unformed body; all the days ordained for me were written in your book before one of them came to be.*

**Romans 8:28**

*And we know that for those who love God all things work together for good, for those who are called according to his purpose.*

**1 Peter 5:10**

*And after you have suffered a little while, the God of all grace, who has called you to his eternal glory in Christ, will himself restore, confirm, strengthen, and establish you.*

**James 1:12**

*Blessed is the man who remains steadfast under trial, for when he has stood the test he will receive the crown of life, which God has promised to those who love him.*

**1 Corinthians 1:9**

*God is faithful, by whom you were called into the fellowship of his Son, Jesus Christ our Lord.*

# He is Faithful

This is the day that the Lord has made. It was never promised to me, so I will rejoice and be glad in it, regardless of my circumstances.

I am reminded that there is nothing in all of life that surprises God. He is able to work all things together for my good, and because I know that, I can be content, and at peace wherever I am; because, He who is faithful gives me the strength to do so. Praise His holy name.

## Today's Readings

**Psalm 118:24**
> *The Lord has done it this very day; let us rejoice today and be glad.*

**Romans 8:28**
> *And we know that for those who love God all things work together for good, for those who are called according to his purpose*

**Philippians 4:11-13**
> *I am not saying this because I am in need, for I have learned to be content whatever the circumstances. I know what it is to be in need, and I know what it is to have plenty. I have learned the secret of being content in any and every situation, whether well fed or hungry, whether living in plenty or in want. I can do all this through him who gives me strength.*

**Matthew 6:31-34**

*Therefore do not be anxious, saying, 'What shall we eat?' or 'What shall we drink?' or 'What shall we wear?' For the Gentiles seek after all these things, and your heavenly Father knows that you need them all. But seek first the kingdom of God and his righteousness, and all these things will be added to you. "Therefore do not be anxious about tomorrow, for tomorrow will be anxious for itself. Sufficient for the day is its own trouble.*

www.ingramcontent.com/pod-product-compliance
Lightning Source LLC
Chambersburg PA
CBHW030530290526
45786CB00004B/1674